I0700918

CHAIR YOGA FOR SENIORS

Gentle Exercise at Home for Holistic Health and Wellness Enhance Flexibility, Improve Balance, and Boost Overall Well-being

CHAIR YOGA FOR SENIORS

Copyright: © 2023 Ruth Gonzalez

All rights reserved. No part of this book may be reproduced or transmitted in any form or by any means, electronic or mechanical, including photocopying, recording, or by any information storage and retrieval system, without permission in writing from the publisher.

TABLE OF CONTENT

INTRODUCTION

Welcome and thank you for joining me on this revolutionary path of health and well-being with Chair Yoga for Seniors. I'm Ruth Gonzalez, a dedicated professional instructor who is enthusiastic about helping older people rediscover their vitality and joy through the gentle yet powerful practice of chair yoga.

In today's fast-paced society, it is vital to address the special needs of seniors, many of whom may have physical restrictions. Chair yoga is a personalized solution that provides a holistic approach to wellness by blending the ancient knowledge of yoga with the convenience of a seated practice.

As an experienced instructor, my goal is to establish a secure and welcoming environment in which elders can start on a refreshing journey that transcends the limitations of age. Chair yoga is a mild beginning or reintroduction to physical activity that focuses on building flexibility, strength, and balance while in the comfort and support of a chair.

Throughout our sessions, we will practice a variety of motions and postures that are specifically designed to improve mobility and eliminate stiffness. The practice goes beyond the physical, incorporating breathwork and mindfulness to improve mental clarity and emotional well-being. We hope to improve overall health and resilience by cultivating a sense of connection among the mind, body, and spirit.

CHAIR YOGA FOR SENIORS

Each session is meticulously planned, taking into account our senior participants' unique requirements and abilities. Whether you're a seasoned yogi or new to the practice, Chair Yoga for Seniors is suitable for all fitness levels. Together, we will create a supportive community that fosters growth, friendship, and a revitalized sense of purpose.

I encourage you to join me on this enlightening trip, where we will not only find the vitality within ourselves, but also celebrate the power and wisdom that comes with age. Let us embrace the transformational potential of Chair Yoga for Seniors and cultivate a healthier, more vibrant lifestyle.

CHAPTER ONE

WHY CHAIR YOGA

Numerous studies have shown that yoga improves one's balance, strength, and stability. Our balance, strength, and stability decline as we age. These three losses are the primary causes of the increase in falls among elderly. Yoga practice might not only slow down but even reverse the tendency of weight loss.

Yoga is actually for people of all ages and abilities. Yoga will help you stay strong and healthy if you are already strong and healthy.
If you have temporary or chronic health concerns, a gentle yoga practice will help you regain some of the strength and flexibility that has been impaired by your condition.

Traditional yoga, on the other hand, can be intimidating for anyone who is not as steady on their feet as they once were, for those who want to start slowly, or for anyone who would feel more confident sitting down. Bring on the chair! While seated, you can reap all of the advantages of yoga. Chair yoga provides all of the same benefits as conventional yoga, such as stress, pain, and tiredness relief, but it can also aid with joint lubrication, balance, and arthritis.

One of the primary goals of yoga is to restore and maintain spinal health. Every component of our body functions improperly when we have bad posture. Breathing and blood flow are restricted by a rounded back. Yoga can help you improve your posture by extending and strengthening your spine.

Another significant advantage of yoga is the emphasis it places on the feet. The cornerstone of your movement is your feet. Most seniors endure occasional or chronic foot discomfort or numbness as a result of years of wear and tear. This can result in reduced movement, which is frequently a cause of falls. Traditional yoga is performed barefoot and works the foot throughout the workout. In all of the workouts, I have placed a strong emphasis on foot stretching and strengthening.

In my practice, I've developed simple chair yoga routines for people of all fitness levels and experience. Many of them are included in this book. My wish is that you would commit to making any routine you begin a habit. To be effective, a regular practice of anything must be both pleasurable and simple to implement!

CHAPTER TWO

SIMPLE TO DO AT HOME

WHAT DO I NEED?

If you're taking the basic program, the only thing you'll need is a straight-backed, non-cushioned chair. It can have arms or not. A folding chair or a kitchen table chair is great. If you need a wheelchair, you are fine.

When you are ready to progress to the intermediate routines, you will need a pair of two-pound dumbbells. These can be purchased at any sporting goods store or online.

WHERE SHOULD I SET UP?

I urge that you establish an environment that you will want to return to. You don't need much space, but I do recommend that you select an uncluttered area in your home. Too many visual distractions will prohibit you from enjoying a tranquil habit.

I strongly advise you to position the chair in front of a mirror.

This will provide you immediate feedback on how you're doing with the positions. Not absolutely necessary, but extremely beneficial.

WHAT SHOULD I WEAR?

Dress in loose, comfortable clothing that does not restrict your movement. If you feel comfortable going barefoot, go ahead and do so. If you like the security of a shoe, wear anything with a rubber sole. On a hard-wood floor, do not wear simply socks. That will make it too slick! Socks are acceptable if you are training on a rug.

HOW SHOULD I PREPARE?

It is usually a good idea to drink water before and after exercising. Seniors are renowned for drinking insufficient water and being dehydrated. Eat nothing for an hour before you begin.
You will be more comfortable if you do not have a full stomach.

WHAT TIME OF DAY IS BEST?

This is entirely up to you and your personal preferences. When do you feel the most energised? I recommend the morning, but everyone has their own body clock. Consistency is more important than time of day. Choose an appropriate time and stick to it. According to research, doing something at the same time every day increases the likelihood of it becoming a habit.

BEYOND THE ESSENTIALS

I am so convinced that you will embrace this program and make it a part of your everyday life that I am going to recommend ways to make this experience more enjoyable. Let us begin with **music!** Music makes us feel wonderful. It makes chores appear less like labor and more like play.

But, regardless of how you listen to music, whether through the radio, a CD player, or your phone, please choose something you appreciate.

Select something that makes you happy. I have a chair yoga client who insists on listening to La Traviata exclusively, and another who requests Pete Seeger. Consider this carefully and choose what is best for you.

WHICH PROGRAM SHOULD I CHOOSE? AND HOW OFTEN SHOULD I DO IT?

The answer may or may not be evident. If it isn't, let's find the best one for you.

If you've never exercised before or haven't done so in a long time, I recommend starting with the novice twenty-minute program.

If you have previously exercised frequently but are currently experiencing physical problems such as a chronic condition, recent surgery, or breathing difficulty, then begin at the beginning. The twenty-minute starter workout is moderate but thorough. Every portion of the body is exercised. You are unlikely to feel sore the next day. If you can commit to doing it every other day, I guarantee you will notice a difference after two weeks.

I am confident that if you follow my advice of having an uncluttered, tranquil space in your house to practise, wearing comfortable attire, and listening to music that makes you feel good, you will not consider four times a week to be excessive.
After three or four weeks, consider increasing your commitment to the thirty-minute starter program. If you believe that the twenty-minute starter routine has gotten too simple, consider trying out the intermediate twenty-minute program.

What if you wish to skip the beginner program entirely and start with the intermediate twenty-minute session? Then I wholeheartedly commend your zeal. If you are an energetic individual who does not have any restricted medical problems but has yet to commit to a regular exercise habit, then hop in! Nothing ventured, nothing gained, as the saying goes. If it proves too difficult, you may always backtrack, begin at the beginning, and gradually but steadily work your way up. The most important thing is that you have chosen to read this book because you want to live a better, happier, and less worried life.
If you received this book as a gift and are reading it to avoid appearing ungrateful, I accept the duty of earning your faith that this is the proper path to take.

CHAIR YOGA FOR SENIORS

CHAPTER THREE

WARMING UP

I always start every practice with five minutes of mild warm-ups. Warm-ups prepare our body to stretch and our muscles to lengthen, which aids in injury prevention. The breath is a vital component of the warm-up. We humans, of course, are always breathing. We don't need to think about it at all to accomplish it.

What I'm referring to here is mindful breathing, in which you take control of it to relax yourself and help you move with ease. I've heard yoga teachers define the attentive breath as the difference between exercise and yoga. I appreciate that this is a tough idea to grasp at first, but I am convinced that once you are comfortable with the routines in this book, you will comprehend and accept the function of the breath. It is our strength, our relaxation, and our guardian.

CHAIR YOGA FOR SENIORS

1. Seated Neck Stretches

- Sit comfortably in your chair with your spine straight.
- Gently tilt your head to one side, bringing your ear closer to your shoulder. Hold it for a few seconds.
- Do the same thing on the other side.
- Rotate your neck gently clockwise and counterclockwise.

2. Shoulder Rolls

- Sit up straight and relax your shoulders.
- Roll your shoulders forward in a circular motion for around 10-15 seconds.
- Switch directions and rotate your shoulders backward for another 10-15 seconds.

3. Wrist and Hand Exercises

- Extend your arms straight in front of you.
- Rotate your wrists clockwise, then counterclockwise.
- Make fists, then open your hands wide, continuing for 10-15 seconds.

4. Seated Cat-Cow Stretch

- Sit near the front of your chair, with your feet flat on the floor.
- Exhale as you arch your back, elevate your chest, and roll your shoulders back (Cow Pose).

Exhale as you circle your back, tucking your chin to your chest (Cat Pose).
- Do this for 1-2 minutes.

5. Seated Forward Bend
- Sit on the edge of your chair, feet flat on the floor.
- Inhale as you stretch your spine, and exhale as you hinge at your hips and reach forward to your toes.
- Hold for 15-30 seconds while breathing deeply.

6. Ankle Circles
- Lift one foot off the floor and rotate your ankle clockwise and then counterclockwise.
- Do the same with the opposite foot.

7. Deep Breathing
- Sit comfortably, close your eyes, and take slow, deep breaths.
- Breathe in via your nose, expanding your abdomen, and exhale through your mouth.
- Pay attention to relaxing your body and emptying your mind.

CHAIR YOGA FOR SENIORS

CHAPTER FOUR

BEGINNER'S 20-MINUTE PROGRAM

You have selected to begin your chair yoga program with a twenty-minute beginner session. Congratulations. I'm glad you're trying this out!

I told you that you wouldn't dislike this.

I'll repeat the warm-up instructions here to avoid having to go to the book repeatedly. Remember my commitment to you, the reader. The following guide is simple, easy to read, and understand.

1. THE BREATH

- Inhale slowly through your nose and exhale slowly through your mouth.
- Avoid forcing the breath.
- Try to keep the exhale as long as the inhale.
- Start with a count of two on the inhale and exhale.
- Consider increasing the length of your inhale and exhale to three to four counts.
- Take four whole breaths.

- Remember to proceed slowly and steadily.

Benefits: This breathing technique promotes relaxation and reduces anxiety. It prepares your body to move.

2. SIDE-NECK BEND

- Start in Mountain Pose.
- Inhale and sit tall.
- Exhale while lowering your right ear to your shoulder.
- Maintain a relaxed shoulder position.
- Inhale to return your head to normal.
- Inhale to sit tall, then exhale to bring your left ear to your left shoulder.
- Inhale to return your head to normal.

That was one set, repeat 3 times each.

Benefits: Stretches the sides of your neck.

3. NECK TURNS

- Return to Mountain Pose.
- On an inhalation, slowly turn your head to the right.
- Exhale slowly and return to the centre.
- Inhale and slowly turn your head to the left.
- Exhale slowly and steadily, then return to the centre.

Repeat 3 times each.

Benefits: Reduces neck stress and improves mobility in the upper back.

4.SHOULDER SHRUGS

- Return to Mountain Pose.
- Inhale and raise your shoulders to your ears, then exhale and return to neutral position.
- Exaggerate the lift.

Repeat 5 times.

Benefits: Reduces muscle tension in the neck and shoulders.

5. WRIST CIRCLES

- Sit tall in Mountain Pose.
- Sit with your tummy to the spine and lift your head to the ceiling.
- Move with your elbows near to your sides and hands extended in front of you.
- Extend your fingers and roll them at the wrists.
- Wiggle your fingers and roll your wrists.
- Roll your wrists ten times, then swap directions and roll another ten times.

Benefits: Warming wrists and fingers. Also reduces inflammation in the hand joints.

6. ARM RAISES WITH BOTH ARMS

- Assume Mountain Pose.
- Take a calm, steady inhale and raise both arms above your head.
- Exhale slowly and steadily, then lower your arms to the beginning position.
- Keep your shoulders relaxed while moving.
- If raising your arms overhead is unpleasant, try raising them to a comfortable level for you.

Do this 5 times.

Benefits: Improves shoulder mobility and strengthens arms.

7. KNEE SWINGS

- Begin by sitting tall in Mountain Pose, belly in and shoulders back.
- Place your hands under your right knee.
- Sit upright with a straight spine.
- Begin by gripping under your knee and kicking your leg back and forth.
- This is one of the quick poses.
- If you can't reach under your knee, sit back in your chair and swing your right leg back and forth with as much speed as comfortable.

Perform 20 times per leg.

Benefits: Improves mobility and range of motion in the knees.

8. ANKLE CIRCLES FOR BOTH LEGS

- Assume Mountain Pose.
- Inhale, elevate your spine and stretch your legs.
- To attain this stance, sit all the way back in your chair.
- Keep your legs straight and rotate your feet and ankles clockwise.
- The only moving body parts are your feet and ankles.

Repeat 10 rotations in each direction.

Benefits: Improves ankle and foot mobility.

9. SHOULDER ROLLS.

- Sit tall in Mountain Pose.
- Inhale as you pull your shoulders up and back, then exhale to return to the beginning position.
- Create a smooth movement in a continuous circle.
- After five calm and steady circles, reverse the direction.
- Inhale, lift your shoulders to the front of your body, then exhale and return to the starting position.
- This direction has always felt odd. Don't worry, you're doing it right!

Perform the movement 5 times in each direction.

Benefits: Increases shoulder joint mobility.

10 .FORWARD BEND WITH STRAIGHT BACK

- Sit upright in your chair, palms resting on your thighs.
- Inhale and bend forward from the hips, leading with your chin.
- Keep your spine straight.
- Go as far as you can with your back straight.
- The bend originates from the hips.
- Exhale and use your hands on your legs to push yourself back up.
- Maintain a straight line of sight during the movement.
- Don't glance down. Depending on your spine's flexibility, the movement may be minimal. That is completely OK.
- Remember the movement is gradual!

Perform each set 5 times.

Benefits: Improves lower back strength and mobility.

11. ALTERNATING ARM RAISES

- Assume Mountain Pose.
- Inhale and elevate your right arm above your head, but only if pain-free.
- If not, raise your arm to a comfortable height.
- Maintain a relaxed shoulder and straight extended arm.
- Exhale and lower your arm down.
- Imagine sliding your arm through water.
- This graphic will help you move your arm more slowly. Switch sides.

Repeat 5 times per side.

Benefits: It lubricates the shoulder joint.

12. TORSO TWIST ARMS UP

- Sit tall in Mountain Pose. Draw your belly in.
- Roll your shoulders up, back, and down your spine.
- Inhale and elevate both arms as far as comfortable.
- Shoulders relaxed. Exhale.
- As you inhale, shift your upper body to the right.
- Maintain a forward-facing posture with raised arms.
- Your head shifts in the direction of the twist.
- On the exhale, return to center.
- Keep your arms raised.
- Inhale and twist your torso to the left.

- Exhale and return to the center.
- After each set, bring your hands back to your lap.

Repeat each set of twists (a right and a left twist) 5 times.

Benefits: Reduces love handles and increases spinal flexibility.

Let us halt here for three full breaths. Inhale slowly and steadily through your nose, then exhale slowly and steadily through your mouth. Try to close your eyes during our breathing breaks. It relieves tension.

13. TORSO TWIST WITH ARMS EXTENDED OUT TO THE SIDES

- Torso twist, arms extended to the sides.
- Take the Mountain Pose.
- On an inhale, stretch your arms out to the sides.
- Exhale.
- On an inhalation, slowly twist to the right.
- Move your head with your outstretched right arm.
- Exhale and return to neutral.
- Do not drop your arms.
- When utilizing a mirror, ensure that your extended arms are even and shoulders are down.
- Inhale and twist to the left.
- Your head moves with your left arm.
- Exhale and lower your arms, resting your hands on your legs.

Perform each set of twists 5 times. Maintain an extended arm position throughout.

Benefits: Tightens the waist and strengthens arms.

14. SIDE LEAN WITH BOTH ARMS UP

- Sit up tall in Mountain Pose.
- Inhale as you raise both arms and stay.
- Eg: Hale.
- On your next breath, lean to the right.
- Exhale and raise your arms back to neutral.
- Lean to the left while inhaling slowly and steadily.
- Keep your arms up over your head.
- Exhale and lift both arms overhead.
- Maintain a relaxed posture with shoulders not bent toward the ears.

Perform 5 sets. The arms remain raised during the exercise.

Benefits: Reduces belly fat.

16. SINGLE ARM AND LEG RAISES

- Assume the mountain pose.
- Inhale and lift your right arm and leg slowly and steadily.
- Exhale and slowly lower your arms and legs.
- Repeat five times on the right side.
- Switch sides and repeat five times on the left side.

Benefits: Strengthens arm and leg muscles. Encourages coordination.

17. SINGLE LEG RAISES

- Sit tall in Mountain Pose.
- Inhale as you lift your right leg from a bent position, then exhale as you return to Mountain Pose.
- Switch sides.
- This is a slow, controlled movement.

Repeat 8 times per side.

Benefits: Improves knee mobility.

18. SINGLE KNEE RAISES

- Sit tall in Mountain Pose.
- slowly lift your right knee straight up and lower your foot to the floor.
- Raise your knee as high as you can.

Repeat 10 times on each side.

Benefits: Strengthens the quadriceps.

19. SINGLE LEG POINT AND FLEX

- Sit up straight in your chair.
- Inhale and stretch your right leg straight in front of you.
- Keep your leg in this posture and point and flex your right foot.
- This can be completed slowly or fast.
- Either way, your foot and ankle receive a great workout.
- Place your hands in a comfortable position, such as on your lap or by your sides. Exaggerate the point and flex.
- When finished, place your foot on the floor and switch sides.

Repeat 15 times on each side.

Benefits: Stretches the shin and calf muscles while strengthening the foot and ankle.

20. TOE SQUEEZE OR TOE SPREAD

- Begin by sitting in the Mountain Pose.
- On an inhale, stretch both legs out in front.
- Hold your toes in place and compress them hard.
- Then, relax the pressure and spread your toes as wide as possible.
- Continue to tighten everything.
- Then release and spread.
- Imagine spreading your toes so far apart that no toes touch.
- This is simply a goal to work for. Typically, one or two toes will come into contact.

Do this at least 15 times. It feels great!

Benefits: Stretches the toes, feet, and ankles.

30

CHAPTER FIVE

INTERMEDIATE 20-MINUTE PROGRAM

Whether you're new to the intermediate level or have graduated from the basic program, I welcome you to this new level of dedication. This routine aims to raise the difficulty of the moves while remaining safe and manageable. Only two two-pound dumbbells are required as new equipment.

After a few months of exercising three to five times per week, many of my students progress from using two-pound weights to three- or even four-pound weights. Save this information for future use.

started checklist:
- Take a glass of water.
- Be comfortable when dressing.
- Make sure your favorite music is ready.
- Position your chair in a tidy area.

- Wear barefoot or rubber-soled shoes on all surfaces. Socks should only be worn on carpet.
- Place this book on a music stand. Keep the book at eye level and dumbbells within easy reach for optimal results.

1. MOUNTAIN POSE

- Sit tall in your chair, with knees hip distance apart and toes pointed straight ahead.
- Rest your hands on your thighs.
- Roll your shoulders up and down, pulling your navel to your spine.

2. THE BREATHE

- Begin by sitting in Mountain Pose.
- Inhale slowly through your nose, then exhale slowly through your mouth.
- Avoid forcing a breath.
- Make the exhalation last as long as the inhale.
- Begin with a count of two on both inhale and exhale.
- Consider lengthening your inhale and exhale to three to four counts.
- Take four full breaths in a row.
- Maintain a calm and steady pace.

Benefits: this breathing technique includes reduced anxiety and calming of the nervous system. It enables your body to move.

CHAIR YOGA FOR SENIORS

3. SIDE NECK BEND

- Come to Mountain Pose as your starting position.
- Inhale to sit up straight.
- Exhale by dropping your right ear to your right shoulder.
- Remember to relax your shoulders.
- Inhale to return your head to balance.
- Inhale and sit tall, then exhale and bring your left ear to your left shoulder.
- Inhale to return your head to balance.

That is only one set.
The set should be repeated 3 times.
Benefits: Stretches the neck's sides.

4. NECK TURNS

- Return to Mountain Pose as the starting position.
- Inhale slowly and turn your head to the right.
- Return to the center slowly as you exhale.
- Inhale slowly and turn your head to the left.
- Return to the center with a slow and steady exhale.

The set should be repeated 3 times.
Benefits: reduced neck stress and improved upper back mobility.

5. SHOULDER SHRUGS

- Return to Mountain Pose.
- Inhale and raise both shoulders to your ears, then exhale and return to neutral.
- Exaggerate lift.

Repeat 5 times.

Benefit: Reduces muscle tension in the neck and shoulders.

6. WRIST CIRCLES

- Sit tall in Mountain Pose.
- Sit with your belly to the spine and your head up to the ceiling.
- To move, keep your elbows tight to your sides and your hands extended in front of you.
- Roll your wrists while keeping your fingers outstretched.
- Wiggle your fingers while rolling your wrists.
- Roll your wrists ten times, then switch direction and repeat ten times.

Benefits: Warms up the wrists and fingertips. Also reduces inflammation in hand joints.

7. RAISES BOTH ARMS

- Assume the Mountain Pose.
- Inhale slowly and steadily, then raise both arms above your head.
- Lower your arms to the beginning position while exhaling slowly and steadily.
- Maintain a relaxed shoulder position when moving.
- If raising your arms aloft is bothersome, adjust the height to your comfort level.

Perform this 5 times.

Benefits: Improves shoulder mobility and arm strength.

8. KNEE SWINGS

- Begin in Mountain Pose by sitting tall, tummy in, shoulders back.
- Clasp your hands below your right knee.
- Maintain a tall and straight posture while sitting.
- Begin by holding your knee and kicking your leg back and forth.
- This stance is quick to do.
- If you can't reach under your knees, sit back in your chair and swing your right leg as fast as you can.

Perform 20 times for each leg.

Benefits: Improves knee mobility and range of motion.

9. SHOULDER SHRUGS

- Begin in a resume mountain pose.
- Inhale as you pull both shoulders up to your ears, then exhale as you return to neutral.
- Exaggerate your lift.

Repeat 5 times.

Benefit: Reduces muscle tension in the neck and shoulders.

10 ANKLE CIRCLES WITH BOTH LEGS

- Start in Mountain Pose.
- Inhale and elevate your spine, extending both legs.
- To attain this stance, recline your chair completely.
- Begin by rotating your feet and ankles clockwise while keeping your legs straight.
- Only your feet and ankles move.

Rotate 10 times in each direction.

Benefits: Allows for greater ankle and foot movement.

11. HANDS ON SHOULDER ROLLS

- Begin in mountain pose.
- Begin by placing your hands on your shoulders and moving in broad circles, beginning with your elbows.
- Breathe easily as you go.
- Change the orientation of your circles.

Repeat 8 times in each direction.

Benefits: Promotes upper-back warmth and relieves neck stress.

12. SHOULDER ROLLS

- Sit tall in Mountain Pose.
- Inhale as you lift your shoulders up and back, then exhale as you return to your starting position.
- Aim for a smooth, continuous circle movement.
- After five calm, steady circles, reverse the motion.
- Inhale, raise your shoulders to the front of your body, then exhale and return to your starting posture.
- This path always feels weird. Don't worry, you're doing it correctly.

Repeat the movement 8 times in each direction.

Benefits: Increases shoulder mobility and flexibility.

13. FORWARD BEND WITH A STRAIGHT BACK

- Sit tall in your chair, palms resting on thighs.
- On an inhale, bend forward from the hips, leading with the chin.
- Keep your back straight.
- Maintain a straight back and only move as far as possible.
- The bend comes from the hips.
- Exhale and push yourself back up with your hands on your legs.
- During movement, maintain a straight ahead gaze.
- Do not look down. Depending on your spine's flexibility, this movement could be minor.
- That is perfectly OK. Remember, the movement is slow.

Repeat 8 times. On the eighth rep, retain a bending position and take a complete breath, inhaling slowly and exhaling slowly. Revert to neutral.

Benefits: Improves lower back mobility and strength.

14. ALTERNATING ARM RAISES WITH WEIGHTS

- Begin in Mountain Pose, holding two-pound weights against your thighs.
- Inhale and elevate your right arm above your head, but only if pain-free.
- If not, raise your arm to a comfortable height.
- Maintain a relaxed shoulder and straight extended arm.
- Exhale and lower your arm down.
- Switch sides.

Repeat 6 times per side. Hold the stance on the last rep of each side and take a big breath. Release the stance and return to neutral. During the exercise, you grip the weights with both hands.

Benefits: lubricating the shoulder joint and strengthening the arms.

15. TORSO TWISTS WITH EXTENDED ARMS AND WEIGHTS

- Assume the Mountain Pose, holding weights in each hand.
- Hold a weight in each hand and extend your arms out to the sides while inhaling.
- Exhale. Inhale and slowly twist to your right.
- Your head moves with your outstretched right arm.
- Exhale and return to neutral.

- Do not drop your arms. When utilizing a mirror, ensure your extended arms are even and shoulders are down.
- Inhale and twist to the left.
- Your head moves with your left arm.
- Return to neutral and lower your arms, placing your hands on your legs.

Repeat each set 8 times. Hold the stance on the last rep of each side and take a big breath. Release the stance and return to neutral.

Benefits: toning the midriff and strengthening the arms.

Let's pause for three full breaths. Inhale slowly and steadily through your nose, then exhale slowly through your mouth.

16. SIDE BODY LEAN WITH WEIGHT

- Sit up tall in Mountain Pose.
- Hold weights in both hands and rest them on your thighs.
- Inhale and push your arms up while holding weights in both hands.
- Exhale. Lean to the right with your next breath.

- Exhale as you raise your arms back to neutral.
- Lean to the left while inhaling slowly and steadily, keeping your arms up over your head.
- Exhale as you raise both arms back overhead.

Perform 8 sets. Arms remain up throughout. On the final rep of each side, hold the pose and take a complete breath.

Release the stance and return to neutral.

Benefits: toned waistline.

17 .BICEP CURLS ALTERNATING ARMS WITH WEIGHTS

- Begin with sitting in Mountain Pose with weights in hand.
- Drop your arms to your sides.
- Hold your elbows to the sides of your body.
- Inhale and slowly bend your right arm up, then exhale and drop it to the beginning position.
- Inhale and raise your left arm, then exhale to return to the starting position.
- Your elbows do not leave the sides of your torso During the movement.

Repeat 8 times per side. Repeat the exercise for eight reps on each side, pausing to take a breath.

Benefit: Increases biceps muscle mass.

18. SINGLE ARM AND LEG RAISE WITH WEIGHTS

- Begin in Mountain Pose, with weights on your lap.
- Inhale and lift your right arm (weight in hand) and right leg together.
- Maintain the straightest possible arm and leg positions.
- Exhale while lowering them.

Repeat 6 times on each side. On the last rep of each side, take a full breath (inhale and exhale) while holding the pose up. Return to neutral position by releasing the stance.

Benefits: increased arm and leg muscle strength. Increases coordination.

19. SINGLE-KNEE RAISES WITH WEIGHTS

- Begin in Mountain Pose, sitting erect and resting both weights on the top of your right knee.
- To do the movement, place your right hand on the two weights and carefully pull your right knee straight up before slowly lowering your foot to the floor.
- For the final rep, raise your knees and take a deep breath. Switch sides after returning

your foot to the floor. Place two weights on top of your left knee.

Repeat 10 times on each side. Take a big breath on the final rep of each half. Hold a release pose.

Benefits: increased quadriceps strength.

20. SIT TO STAND

- Sit tall in your seat.
- Place your hands on the sides of the chair's seat. Bend gently forward, keeping your back straight and looking straight ahead.
- Lift up six inches off the chair and return to a sitting position.

Repeat the movement 8 times. Extend your arms straight out in front of you as you get out of the chair.

Benefits: Strengthens the gluteus muscles responsible for sitting and standing. Improving overall equilibrium.

CHAIR YOGA FOR SENIORS

CHAPTER SIX

ADVANCED 30-MINUTE PROGRAM

This routine requires only three- and four-pound weights. This regimen focuses on gaining and maintaining muscle strength, unlike beginner and intermediate programs. Always feel free to make modifications. By this point in your yoga journey, you've gained a better understanding of your body's limitations. Listen to it.

Start your workout with five minutes of warm-ups, as usual.

When your warm-up is over, you can begin. Keep the three- and four-pound weights close by hand. Remember to stay hydrated both before and after exercise.

1. MOUNTAIN POSE

- Sit tall in your chair, knees comfortably hip distance apart, and toes pointed straight front.
- Put your hands on your thighs.

- Roll your shoulders up and down your back, pulling your navel to your spine.

2. THE BREATH

- Sit in Mountain Pose.
- Inhale slowly and steadily through your nose, then exhale slowly through your mouth.
- Don't force your breath. Try to make the exhale as long as the inhalation.
- Begin with a two-count inhalation and exhalation. Consider taking lengthier inhale and exhale counts, such as three to four.

Take four full breaths. Remember to go slowly and steadily.

Benefits: This breathing technique relaxes the nervous system and relieves anxiety. It prepares your body for movement.

3. SIDE NECK BEND

- Assume Mountain Pose.
- Inhale to sit upright.
- Exhale while lowering your right ear to your right shoulder.
- Make sure your shoulders are relaxed.
- Inhale to bring your head back into neutral. Inhale to sit tall, then exhale while bringing your left ear to your left shoulder.
- Inhale to bring your head back into neutral.

- That's one set.

Repeat the set 3 times.

Benefits: It stretches the sides of the neck.

4. NECK TURNS

- Return to Mountain Pose.
- Inhale and slowly turn your head to the right.
- As you exhale, slowly return to the center. As you inhale, slowly turn your head to the left.
- Exhale slowly and steadily, then return to center position.

Repeat the set 3 times.

Benefits: Reduces neck stress and improves mobility in the upper back.

5. SHOULDER SHRUGS

- Return to Mountain Pose.
- Inhale and raise your shoulders to your ears, then exhale and return to neutral position.
- Exaggerate the lift.

Repeat 5 times.

Benefits: Reduces muscle tension in the neck and shoulders.

6. WRIST CIRCLES
- Sit tall in Mountain Pose.
- Sit with your tummy to the spine and lift your head to the ceiling.
- Move with your elbows near to your sides and hands extended in front of you.
- Extend your fingers and roll them at the wrists.
- Wiggle your fingers and roll your wrists.
- Roll your wrists ten times, then swap directions and roll another ten times.

Benefits: Warms the wrists and fingers. Also reduces inflammation in the hand joints.

7. ARM RAISES WITH BOTH ARMS
- Assume Mountain Pose.
- Take a calm, steady inhale and raise both arms above your head.
- Exhale slowly and steadily, then lower your arms to the beginning position.
- Keep your shoulders relaxed while moving.
- If raising your arms overhead is unpleasant, try raising them to a comfortable level for you.

Do this 5 times.

Benefits: Improves shoulder mobility and strengthens arms.

8. KNEE SWINGS

- Begin by sitting tall in Mountain Pose, belly in and shoulders back.
- Movement: Place your hands under your right knee.
- Sit upright with a straight spine.
- Begin by gripping under your knee and kicking your leg back and forth.
- This is one of the quick poses.
- If you can't reach under your knee, sit back in your chair and swing your right leg back and forth with as much speed as comfortable.

Perform 20 times per leg.

Benefits: improved knee mobility and range of motion.

10. ALTERNATING ARM RAISES WITH WEIGHTS

- Begin in Mountain Pose, holding two-pound weights against your thighs.
- Inhale and elevate your right arm above your head, but only if pain-free.
- If not, raise your arm to a comfortable height. Maintain a relaxed shoulder and straight extended arm.

- Exhale and lower your arm down.
- Switch sides.

Repeat 6 times per side. Hold the stance on the last rep of each side and take a big breath. Release the stance and return to neutral. During the exercise, you grip the weights with both hands.

Benefits: lubricating the shoulder joint and strengthening the arms.

Let's pause for three full breaths. Inhale slowly and steadily through your nose, then exhale slowly through your mouth.

11. TORSO TWIST WITH WEIGHTS ON THE SHOULDERS

- Assume the Mountain Pose, holding weights in each hand and placing them on your shoulders.
- On an inhalation, slowly twist to the right.
- Your head moves with your right arm.
- Exhale and return to neutral.
- Do not drop your arms.
- Inhale and twist to the left.
- Your head moves with your left arm.
- Return to neutral and lower your arms, resting them on your legs.

Repeat each set 8 times. Take two full breaths while holding the stance for the last rep on each side. Release the stance and return to neutral.

Benefits: toning the midriff and strengthening the arms.

12. SIDE BODY LEAN WITH WEIGHT

- Sit up tall in Mountain Pose.
- Hold weights in both hands and rest them on your thighs.
- Inhale and push your arms up while holding weights in both hands.
- Exhale.
- Lean to the right with your next breath. Exhale as you raise your arms back to neutral.
- Lean to the left while inhaling slowly and steadily, keeping your arms up over your head.
- Exhale as you lift both arms aloft.

Perform 8 sets. Arms remain up throughout. Hold the posture for two full breaths on each side's final rep. Release the stance and return to neutral.

Benefits: toned waistline.

13. BICEP CURLS WITH ALTERNATING ARMS AND WEIGHTS

- Begin with sitting in Mountain Pose with weights in hand.
- Drop your arms to your sides.
- Hold your elbows to the sides of your body. Inhale and slowly bend your right arm up, then exhale and drop it to the beginning position.
- Inhale and raise your left arm, then exhale to return to the starting position.
- Ensure your elbows remain on the sides of your torso during the action.

Repeat 8 times per side. Repeat the exercise for eight reps on each side, pausing to take a breath.

Benefits: Increases biceps muscle mass.

14. OVERHEAD TRICEPS CURLS WITH WEIGHTS

- Sit in Mountain Pose.
- Hold one weight overhead with both hands and a slight bend in the elbows.
- Inhale.

- Exhale and lower your hands to your upper back, keeping your forearms parallel to the floor and elbows close to your head.
- Inhale and extend your hands back to the overhead position.
- Exhale.

Perform 6 sets of this workout. Return to the resting Mountain Pose. Take two deep breaths and repeat the 6 sets.

Benefits: Strengthens the triceps and upper back.

15. SINGLE ARM AND LEG RAISES WITH WEIGHTS

- Start in Mountain Pose with weights in your lap.
- Inhale and lift your right arm and leg together.
- Maintain maximum straightness in both arms and legs.
- Exhale as you lower them.

Repeat 6 times per side. On the final rep of each side, take two full breaths while holding the pose up. Release the stance and return to neutral.

Benefits: Strengthens arm and leg muscles. Encourages coordination.

CHAIR YOGA FOR SENIORS

16. SINGLE KNEE RAISES WITH WEIGHTS

- Begin by sitting erect in Mountain Pose with both weights resting on the top of your right knee.
- place your right hand on the two weights and slowly pull your right knee straight up before lowering your foot to the floor.
- Repeat ten times.
- For the final rep, raise your knees and take two full breaths.
- Return your foot to the floor and switch sides.
- Position the two weights on top of your left knee.

Repeat 10 times on each side. Take two full breaths during the last rep of each side. Release the position.

Benefits: Strengthens the quadriceps.

17. ADVANCED SIT TO STAND

- Starting Position: Sit tall in your chair.
- Bend forward gently, keeping your back straight and looking straight ahead.
- Extend your arms straight out in front.
- Lift up from your chair, stand tall, and then sit back down.
- Keep your arms extended.

Perform the movement 8 times fast. Repeat eight times gently, taking a breath in between.

Benefits: Increases overall strength, particularly in the gluteus muscles, and improves balance. Also strengthens the core.

18. SINGLE LEG POINT WITH FLEX

- Start by sitting tall in your chair with a straight spine.
- Inhale and straighten your right leg in front of you.
- Begin pointing and flexing your right foot while maintaining your leg stance. This can be done both slowly and quickly. This manner, your feet and ankles get a great workout.
- Place your hands in a comfortable position, such as by your sides or in your lap.
- Exaggerate both the point and the flex. Finish by returning your foot to the floor and switching sides.

Perform 15 times on each side.

Benefits: Stretches shin and calf muscles, strengthens the foot and ankle.

19. SINGLE LEG ANKLE CIRCLES

- Sit tall in your chair, in Mountain Pose.
- Inhale and elevate your right leg.
- Rotate your foot clockwise.
- Gradually articulate the circles.
- Exaggerate their size.
- After about ten rotations, switch directions. Maintain maximum straightness in your elevated leg.
- Switch your legs.

Repeat 10 times on each side.

Benefits: Increases ankle mobility and strength.

20. BENT OVER THE ROW WITH WEIGHTS

- Begin in Mountain Pose, holding weights and resting on your legs.
- Bend forward from the hips, keeping your back straight.
- Look directly forward.
- While inhaling, bring your elbows back and keep your arms close to your sides.
- Exhale slowly, lowering your arms all the way down.
- Maintain a straight arm and forward-bent position.
- As you inhale, carefully pull your arms back up.

- At the apex of the position, your hands should be at the sides of your chest.
- Exhale and lower your arms to the straight posture.
- Maintain a straight back and forward bend during the exercise, looking straight ahead.

Repeat 6 sets, pausing for two full breaths between each.

Benefits: Increases upper and lower back strength, as well as biceps.

CHAPTER SEVEN

I'M FEELING SO MUCH BETTER DO I NEED MORE?

Friends and relatives may have observed changes in you as a result of frequent chair yoga practice.

You feel taller, more confident, have a positive outlook, and breathe more easily. I hope this has left you wanting more. What is there more of? I'll tell you.

Numerous lifestyle modifications can improve happiness, health, and fulfillment. If you want to improve your health, happiness, fulfillment, purpose, and serenity, continue reading this chapter. I hope my experiences can inspire you to broaden your horizons.

If you are willing to investigate, please be patient while I make some assumptions about you. You likely purchased this book hoping to improve your mood. You likely started with the basic routines and acquired confidence and strength to progress to the intermediate section of the book. You've probably included chair yoga into your everyday practice. Set up your home area to work through a 20-30 minute program three times a week. Move your neck, shoulders, legs, and feet wherever you sit. You feel good. Better than you've done in a long time. You experience less tension and stress, and your aches and pains are better managed. Are I describing you? Or perhaps a different version of yourself? If you can relate to these details, you're ready to embrace a holistic and healthy lifestyle.

I will discuss four proven topics that can significantly improve your life.

The four topics that we will explore are:
- The Benefits of Eating healthily.
- The benefits of meditation.
- The benefits of volunteering.
- The importance of community and social connections.

HEALTHY EATING

Let's start with a healthy diet. The media frequently advertises weight-loss regimens. Commercials and content are often difficult to differentiate.

There are meal plans, protein drinks and supplements, as well as eating and fasting instructions provided. It makes you dizzy! I was raised in a traditional Turkish-American household with plenty of food. We encouraged each other to eat. Eating was a social activity. The primary focus is on food. It took me several years to comprehend the importance of eating in my life. I continue to work on it. I keep a healthy weight. But it's not easy for me. When my weight continued to grow, I tried many weight loss methods over time. Maintaining a healthy diet benefited me.

What defines a healthy diet? Experts have regularly endorsed the Mediterranean diet. It is more of a lifestyle than a diet. It's linked to a 25% lower risk of heart disease. It is also widely recommended for people with type 2 diabetes.

What is a Mediterranean diet made of? The diet is plant-based, with protein served as a "side." Eat plenty of vegetables and fruits, avoid skinless chicken and fish, and consume moderate amounts of legumes, nuts, and healthy fats like olive oil and avocado. Sweets and alcohol are allowed in moderation.

MEDITATION

If you have never meditated, you may reject it as a new-age practice that it's not for you. I'd like to dispel common misconceptions about meditation and introduce you to a practice that can improve stress management, reduce blood pressure, and increase peace of mind. This sounds too wonderful to be true. But it's true.

Meditation is a simple practice that allows the brain to relax from the constant stream of ideas. Practicing for just five minutes per day can be useful and easy. Meditation, like exercise, is most effective when practiced regularly. Practicing meditation for five to ten minutes every day can alleviate stress and prevent sadness and insomnia associated with aging.

How do you do this? To begin, adopt a comfortable seating position that supports your back and promotes relaxation. Uncross your legs and arms, then place your hands in your lap. When starting a meditation practice, consider using a timer. Use a kitchen timer, stop watch, or any gadget that can be set for at least five minutes.

Allow your body and mind to relax. Begin by opening your eyes and maintaining a gentle focus. Take deep breaths and slowly close your eyes. Breathe naturally. Pay attention to how your body feels. Start with your head and move down your body. Breathe gently. As you inhale, your abdomen expands and your shoulders relax. Allow yourself to have thoughts. Focus your attention back on your breath. Consider how air enters and exits your body with each inhale and exhale. You can consider the words **"I am breathing in, I am breathing out."** This will help you center yourself and return to your meditation practice. When the time is up, slowly open your eyes and take in the surroundings.

Practicing meditation at the same time every day can help individuals maintain a consistent practice. If this is not feasible for you, schedule a peaceful five to ten minute time slot whenever possible.

To explore different meditation techniques, use the Headspace App on your smartphone or search for guided meditations on YouTube. After chair yoga, it's ideal to meditate immediately. You established the ideal environment for your exercise. It is a really simple transition.

VOLUNTEERING

Volunteering is a strong activity that not only helps communities but also provides countless personal advantages to volunteers. First and foremost, volunteering gives people a sense of purpose and fulfillment. Participating in activities that benefit others or the community as a whole can provide a profound sense of fulfillment while also improving mental and emotional well-being.

Second, volunteering provides an opportunity to learn new skills or improve existing ones. Volunteers frequently gain significant experiences that can benefit both their personal and professional lives, whether they are organizing events, working in a team, or learning specific duties. This constant learning process can be especially advantageous for anyone looking for personal growth or new professional opportunities.

Furthermore, volunteering promotes a sense of belonging and community. Volunteers generate a sense of connection among other participants by working together to achieve common goals. This social aspect is important for mental health since it provides a support network that can be useful during times of personal difficulty.

Additionally, volunteering might have a favorable impact on physical health. Many volunteer activities include physical responsibilities, which promote an active lifestyle. This might be especially useful for those who want to maintain or improve their physical health. Volunteering is a comprehensive approach to overall health since it provides mental, emotional, and physical advantages.

Finally, volunteering can lead to extended networks and opportunities. Volunteers frequently make relationships with broad groups of people, which can lead to new friendships, employment possibilities, and other life-changing events. These increased social networks can have a long-term favorable impact on many elements of one's life.

COMMUNITY AND SOCIAL CONNECTIONS

Community and social relationships are critical for people of all ages, but they are especially important for seniors. One of the key advantages is the improvement of mental and emotional health. Social contacts diminish emotions of isolation and loneliness, two common concerns among the elderly. Being a part of a community gives a support network that improves general happiness and mental health.

Social interactions can improve cognitive performance. Conversations, group activities, and remaining socially active have all been linked to improved cognitive function in seniors. Regular social contacts stimulate the brain, potentially lowering the risk of cognitive decline while increasing mental sharpness.

Furthermore, community involvement helps seniors feel purposeful and relevant. Being actively involved in social and community events provides children something to look forward to every day, which promotes a good attitude on life. This sense of purpose can lead to a better quality of life in their later years.

In addition, social interactions are important for elders' physical health. According to research, those who have strong social support networks are more likely to engage in healthy habits like regular exercise and a good diet. This can lead to improved overall health and longevity.

CHAIR YOGA FOR SENIORS

CONCLUSION

Have you been practicing chair yoga for a while and can't stop talking about it?
I believe the compliments you've received have contributed to your positive outlook. Regular exercise affects our appearance, movement, and communication with others. It promotes relaxation and reduces stress levels. Consistent attentive breathing helps cleanse our mind.

I'm sure you've noticed that I use the word "habit" frequently.
This is not an accident. A habit is something repeated on a regular basis without conscious thought. You are instinctively driven to do it. A habit is not something you do sometimes. A habit can be positive or negative. For most people, smoking is the first unpleasant habit that springs to mind. Good habits include regular exercise, reading, and volunteering. I am sure you can think of many more.

The key to developing the habit is consistency. Practicing chair yoga at least three times a week is a habit. You can also practice positions throughout the day, regardless of where you sit. Consistency is essential.
Now, how does this relate to sharing with friends? After experiencing the benefits of exercise, it's natural to want to share your experience with others. Sharing means more than simply informing

others about your experience and encouraging them to try it. I recommend organizing a small group and meeting in your home or someone else's. How do you do this? Here are some suggestions.

Find a space large enough for a few chairs. For a successful group expedition, start with one or two buddies and grow as needed. Set up chairs in a horseshoe shape. This layout enables for eye contact with one another. Ensure that everyone may stretch their arms and legs freely while seated.

Ideally, each participant should have the Chair Yoga for Seniors book. Otherwise, whoever has the book will read the instructions. After some experience, you may be able to recall the instructions from memory. Avoid revealing too much information to your invited guests, as they will need to know every aspect for perfect execution of the postures.

Agree on what music you will listen to. You and your pals are likely to share similar music choices. Be creative here.

If someone in your group uses Spotify or Apple Music, they can make an entertaining playlist for group sessions.

This should be a fun activity. Set some ground rules, but don't be too strict. Don't worry about the timing. Allow enough time for everyone to learn and execute each posture properly. As you bring this group together, please remember to work within your own range of motion and avoid painful exercises.

Drink a glass of water and begin warm-ups!

YOUR JOURNAL

HABIT TRACKER

Date:______________________

EXERCISE	REPS	SETS	✓
			○
			○
			○
			○
			○
			○
			○
			○
			○
			○

NOTES

HABIT TRACKER

Date: _______________

EXERCISE	REPS	SETS	✓
			○
			○
			○
			○
			○
			○
			○
			○
			○
			○

NOTES

HABIT TRACKER

Date:_______________

EXERCISE	REPS	SETS	

NOTES

HABIT TRACKER

Date: ___________________

EXERCISE	REPS	SETS	⬤
			○
			○
			○
			○
			○
			○
			○
			○
			○
			○

NOTES

HABIT TRACKER

Date: ______________________

EXERCISE	REPS	SETS	✓
			◯
			◯
			◯
			◯
			◯
			◯
			◯
			◯
			◯
			◯

NOTES

HABIT TRACKER

Date:_______________________

EXERCISE	REPS	SETS	○
			○
			○
			○
			○
			○
			○
			○
			○
			○
			○

NOTES

HABIT TRACKER

Date: _______________

EXERCISE	REPS	SETS	⬤
			○
			○
			○
			○
			○
			○
			○
			○
			○
			○

NOTES

HABIT TRACKER

Date: _______________

EXERCISE	REPS	SETS	○
			○
			○
			○
			○
			○
			○
			○
			○
			○
			○

NOTES

HABIT TRACKER

Date: _________________________

EXERCISE	REPS	SETS	✓
			○
			○
			○
			○
			○
			○
			○
			○
			○
			○

NOTES

HABIT TRACKER

Date: ___________________

EXERCISE	REPS	SETS	⬤
			○
			○
			○
			○
			○
			○
			○
			○
			○
			○

NOTES

HABIT TRACKER

Date: _______________

EXERCISE	REPS	SETS	✓
			○
			○
			○
			○
			○
			○
			○
			○
			○
			○

NOTES

HABIT TRACKER

Date: ___________________

EXERCISE	REPS	SETS	○
			○
			○
			○
			○
			○
			○
			○
			○
			○
			○

NOTES

HABIT TRACKER

Date: _______________________

EXERCISE	REPS	SETS	✓
			○
			○
			○
			○
			○
			○
			○
			○
			○
			○

NOTES

HABIT TRACKER

Date: _______________________

EXERCISE	REPS	SETS	⬤
			◯
			◯
			◯
			◯
			◯
			◯
			◯
			◯
			◯
			◯

NOTES

HABIT TRACKER

Date: ______________________

EXERCISE	REPS	SETS	✓
			○
			○
			○
			○
			○
			○
			○
			○
			○
			○

NOTES

www.ingramcontent.com/pod-product-compliance
Lightning Source LLC
Chambersburg PA
CBHW071610270726
48661CB00019B/1944